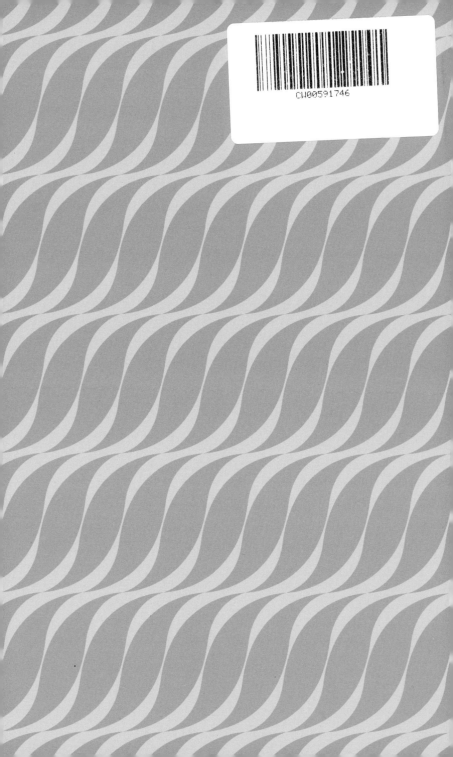

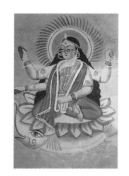

healing with
ayurveda

A concise guide to the ancient
holistic healthcare system

RAJE AIREY

southwater

This edition is published by Southwater

Southwater is an imprint of Anness Publishing Limited,
Hermes House, 88–89 Blackfriars Road, London SE1 8HA
Tel: 020 7401 2077   Fax: 020 7633 9499
info@anness.com

© Anness Publishing Limited 2002

Published in the USA by Southwater
Anness Publishing Inc.
fax: 212 807 6813

This edition distributed in the UK by
The Manning Partnership
tel: 01225 852 727
fax: 01225 852 852
sales@manning-partnership.co.uk

This edition distributed in the USA by
National Book Network
tel: 301 459 3366
fax: 301 459 1705
www.nbnbooks.com

This edition distributed in Canada by
General Publishing
tel. 416 445 3333
fax 416 445 5991
www.genpub.com

This edition distributed in Australia by
Sandstone Publishing
tel: 02 9560 7888
fax: 02 9560 7488
sales@sandstonepublishing.com.au

This edition distributed in New Zealand
by The Five Mile Press (NZ) Ltd
tel: 09 444 4144
fax 09 444 4518
fivemilenz@clear.net.nz

Publisher: Joanna Lorenz
Managing Editor: Helen Sudell
Project Editor: Simona Hill
Designer: Nigel Partridge
Photographers: Peter Anderson, Simon Bottomley,
Martin Brigdale, Jonathan Buckley, Nick Cole,
Nicki Dowey, Gus Filgate, John Freeman,
Michelle Garrett, Christine Hanscomb,
Amanda Heywood, Janine Hosegood,
Alistair Hughes, Andrea Jones, Dave King, Don Last, William Lingwood,
Steve Moss, Thomas Odulate, Debbie Patterson, Anthony Pickhaver,
Fiona Pragoff, Sam Stowell, Mark Wood
Production Controller: Joanna King

Publisher's note: The reader should not regard the recommendations, ideas
and techniques expressed and described in this book as substitutes for the
advice of a qualified medical practitioner or other qualified professional. Any use
to which the recommendations, ideas and techniques is put is at the reader's
sole discretion and risk.

1 3 5 7 9 10 8 6 4 2

contents

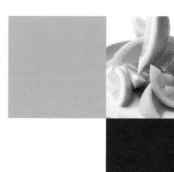

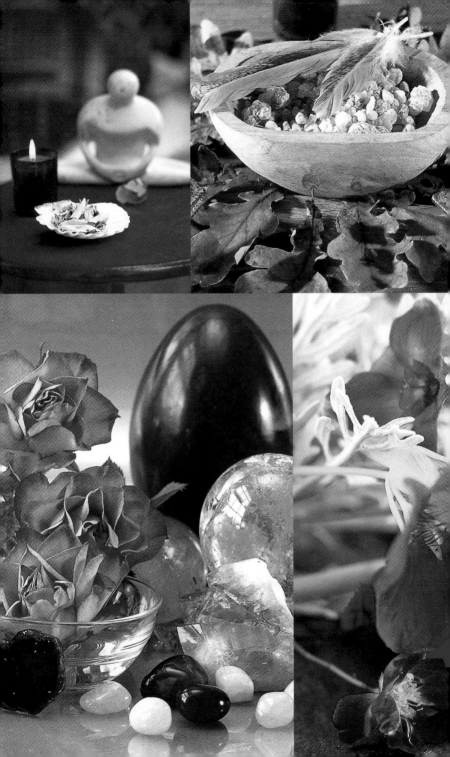

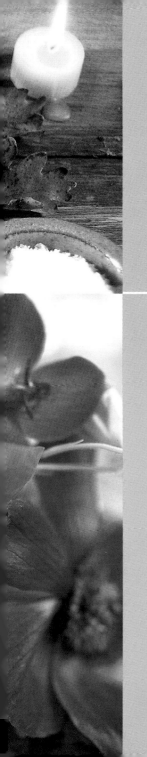

introduction

According to legend, the 52 great Rishis (seers) of ancient India discovered the Veda, or knowledge of how the universe works, in their meditations. These secrets were then organized into a system known as Ayurveda, which means "science of life".

Increasingly popular as a holistic system of healthcare in the Western world, Ayurveda gives clear instructions on how we can achieve physical and spiritual wellbeing. Through the discovery of our constitutional type, known as our dosha, it shows how we can prevent and treat disease by paying attention to diet and lifestyle, and how to strengthen and heal the body using a diversity of techniques, including yoga, colour, crystals, massage and much more.

what is ayurveda?

Ayurveda is the art of living a balanced life. This is the pathway to good health, happiness and longevity, and Ayurveda teaches a broad-based doctrine of holistic living with practical instructions on how we may best achieve this.

Rooted in the philosophical and spiritual traditions of India, at the heart of Ayurveda is the understanding that everything in the universe is interconnected: we are not isolated individuals but are part of the greater whole, linked to the web of life by invisible energy pathways, or prana, the "breath of life". Similarly, within each of us, every-

thing is connected and operating on many different levels. Ayurveda recognizes that our emotions, intellect and physical body, together with our actions and surrounding environment, are all interlinked and influence each other. Good health is achieved when all these aspects are balanced and in proportion with one another. This leads to inner

▼ CRYSTALS HELP TO CHANNEL ENERGY AS PART OF THE AYURVEDIC HEALING PROCESS.

▼ IN AYURVEDA meditation helps to BALANCE THE BODY, MIND AND SPIRIT.

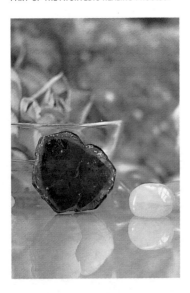

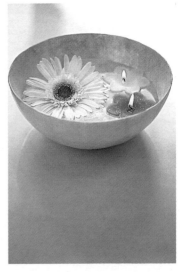

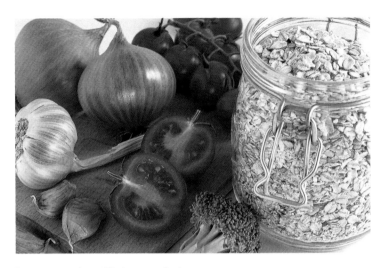

harmony and equilibrium – a feeling of being "at one" with the world and oneself.

There are eight branches to the "tree" of Ayurveda, each one covering various aspects of health and healing, including surgery, gynaecology, paediatrics and medicine. Ayurvedic medicine is the branch responsible for treating our health on a day-to-day basis. Its aim is to prevent and treat ill-health so that we are left free to develop our spiritual potential. This does not mean that you have to have any particular religious belief to benefit from Ayurvedic medicine as the philosophy both acknowledges the uniqueness of the individual, and

▲ Choosing a healthy diet that suits our dosha is the basis of wellbeing.

is also very practical in its applications. It is founded on the belief that all diseases stem from the digestive system and are caused by poor digestion and/or by following an improper diet.

Ayurveda's primary method of treatment is through nutrition, supported by the use of herbs, massage and aromatic oils, but there are also many other complementary branches, including yoga and meditation, crystals and colour healing. It is about finding what works for you and then applying it to improve your life in whatever ways seem most fitting.

elemental energies

Everything in the universe is shaped by the cosmic energies of space (or ether), air, fire, water and earth. These heavenly forces combine into three fundamental life energies, or doshas, of the human body; vata, pitta and kapha.

The elements are graded beginning with ether, the highest, lightest and most rare, followed by air, then fire and water. The density of earth makes it the heaviest element. Each dosha is a combination of two elements, which predisposes them towards certain principles.

Ayurveda recognizes that each individual is a creation of cosmic energies and a unique phenomenon. No other person has an identical dosha pattern to our own. The combination of vata, pitta and kapha in each of us is determined at conception and is influenced by the season, time of day, and the genetics, diet, lifestyle and emotional state of our parents. Some people are born with a constitution in which all three doshas are equally balanced, which suggests exceptionally good health and a long life span.

However, in most of us, one or two doshas predominate. This unique and specific combination of the doshas is referred to as the "prakruti", our basic nature or constitution. As we experience life's ups

▼ ETHER SUGGESTS A LIGHT AND TRANSIENT STATE. THIS IS THE HIGHEST ELEMENT.

▼ AIR IS HEAVIER THAN ETHER, BUT LIGHTER THAN THE OTHER THREE ELEMENTS.

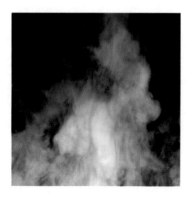

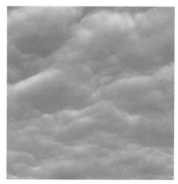

Characteristics of Each Dosha

dosha	element	cosmic link	character	principle	influence
vata	ether/air	wind	dry/cold	change	activity
pitta	fire/water	sun	hot	conversion	metabolism
kapha	water/earth	moon	moist	inertia	cohesion

and downs, the balance of the doshas in our mind-body system changes. The "vikruti" is our current state of health, influenced by such things as our diet, stress levels, emotional state, physical fitness, and even the weather. If your health is excellent, your vikruti and your prakruti may match. Much more likely, however, is that there will be a discrepancy between the two. The aim of Ayurvedic medicine is to re-establish the balance required by your prakruti.

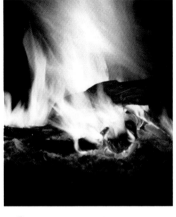

▲ FIRE HAS THE QUALITIES OF HEAT AND DRYNESS. IT IS MIDWAY IN THE ELEMENTS.

▼ WATER SUGGESTS COOL, SMOOTH AND SOFT QUALITIES. IT DESCENDS INTO EARTH.

▼ EARTH IS THE HEAVIEST OF THE FIVE ELEMENTS AND SUGGESTS A SLOW ENERGY.

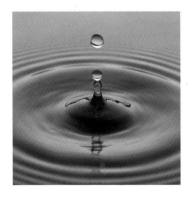

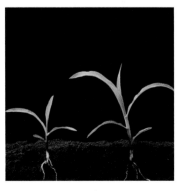

elemental energies **9**

lifestyle influences

The theory of the doshas is central to Ayurvedic medicine. All bodily, mental and spiritual functions are controlled by the vital forces of vata, pitta and kapha. Health is achieved when these forces are working in harmony.

The subtle energies of vata, pitta and kapha cannot be perceived by any of the senses, yet they are thought to move, increase or diminish, and seem invisibly linked. Changes in the balance of one dosha can have a knock-on effect on the others. In fact the word dosha means "that which tends to go out of balance easily".

Imbalance occurs when we go against our own nature (prakruti) over a long period of time. A modern Western lifestyle and living in an urban environment seems to make us particularly susceptible. Eating an unhealthy or unsuitable diet puts the body under stress. We suffer pollution in our food, air and water, and even the medicines we take have potentially harmful side-effects. We overload our senses by spending too much time on noisy, polluted city streets, working

▼ TAKE TIME TO RELAX AND ENJOY THE COMPANY OF FRIENDS.

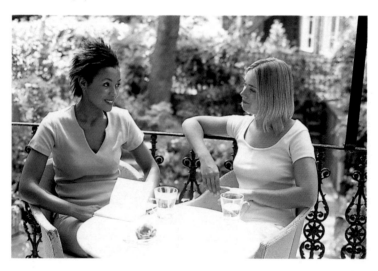

long hours or watching television. There is pressure to live life on the run, eat "fast" food, and overwork in the pursuit of material gain and the realization of goals.

Negative thoughts and emotions affect how we feel, but generally we do not allow ourselves enough time to relax and unwind and to return to mental equilibrium. We tend to forget about the body and its needs and only consider our health when it breaks down and stops us "getting on" with things. When all these factors are taken together, it is hardly surprising that stress-related illnesses are on the increase in the Western world.

However, retreating from life and becoming a hermit is not the answer. Sensory stimulation, desire and challenge are part of life. The approach of Ayurveda is one of balance and it advocates living in tune with nature's laws, paying attention to the rhythms of day and night, the changing seasons and our age. When we get the balance right we live in harmony with our bodies. It is when we go to extremes and pay insufficient attention to the natural patterns of life that we are liable to throw the doshas off balance.

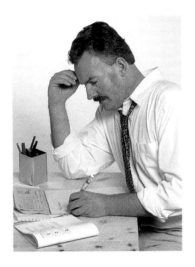

▲ BALANCE YOUR WORKING HOURS WITH RELAXATION, PUTTING THE SAME AMOUNT OF EFFORT INTO EACH.

▼ AYURVEDA TEACHES US TO ATTUNE OUR ATTENTION TO THE NEEDS OF OUR BODIES.

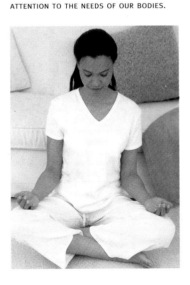

ayurveda & dis-ease

When the doshas are thrown out of balance their energies become over- or under-stimulated, leading to excess or blocked energy in the body. If these imbalances are left untreated, they will eventually manifest as illness.

The purpose of Ayurveda is to recognize the early warning signs of doshic imbalance so as to "catch" the condition and treat the "dis-ease" before it develops into a serious health problem. If the early warning signs, such as mood swings, low energy levels, persistent aches and pains, or poor digestion over a period of time, are ignored then illness will eventually result.

"AMA"

The main effect of imbalance in the doshas is a build-up of "ama" in the body: these are damaging toxins and waste products. A white coating on the tongue is seen as evidence of ama in the body. The aim of Ayurvedic medicine is to deep-cleanse the system (mind and body) of ama and to restore the balance between the doshas.

▼ DRINKING SEVERAL GLASSES OF WATER EVERY DAY HELPS TO FLUSH OUT TOXINS.

▼ MASSAGE HELPS TENSION TO DISPERSE AND IS PLEASANT TO GIVE AND RECEIVE.

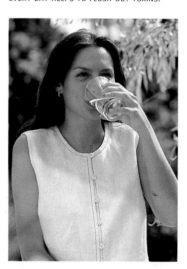

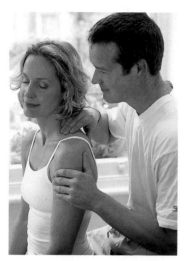

There are many Ayurvedic treatments based on ways to effectively detoxify the system. One simple method is to sip boiled water continuously throughout the day; hot water stimulates the metabolism and encourages the elimination of toxins. Additionally, fasting, eating light meals suitable for your doshic type, meditation and yoga, regular massage and exercise all have a purifying effect on the body and mind. Ayurvedic practitioners advocate moderation in all things to create balance and harmony in the mind and body.

▼ EAT A LIGHT BREAKFAST THAT IS HEALTHY AS WELL AS APPETIZING.

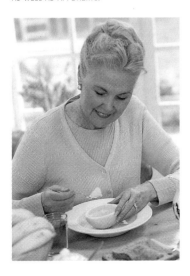

THE SEVEN STAGES TO ILL-HEALTH

Ayurveda sees illness as a gradual process that happens over time and recognizes seven distinct stages. These are states that we are all susceptible to, and some of them are stages that we can actively do something to resolve.

1 Doshic imbalance. This is caused by negative influences, such as poor diet, inadequate rest, environmental pollution or emotional stresses and strains.

2 Aggravation. While the above negative influences continue, the doshas become more seriously unbalanced.

3 Dispersion. The imbalance begins to spread to other parts of the body.

4 Relocation. The affected dosha relocates elsewhere in the body, causing an accumulation of toxic waste products.

5 Mild symptoms. These show in the area where the doshic imbalance is located. It may be at this stage that our attention is brought to our sense of ill-health.

6 Acute illness. In time the symptoms may flare up into an acute condition.

7 Chronic condition. This is the final stage when the symptoms have taken root in the body.

identifying the doshas

Vata, pitta and kapha are associated with psychological and physical characteristics that influence how we look, think, feel and function. Ayurveda uses these distinctions to determine our constitution (prakruti) and state of health (vikruti).

The characteristics of the doshas are influenced by the elemental energies that make them up. Ayurveda recognizes specific states: there are hot and cold people, thin and fat people, dry and moist people. These body types will have different tendencies emotionally, mentally and physically, and therefore will be affected by different types of food and need different approaches to treatment.

Ayurveda stresses the importance of following the correct diet and lifestyle for your dosha. A basic approach to Ayurveda is to first identify your dosha, at the levels of both prakruti and vikruti and then learn how to eat and live in accordance with this information. If the vikruti is different from the prakruti,

you should begin by dealing with the vikruti first, following the guidelines for how to heal your current emotional, physical or mental health conditions with the use of diet and other basic Ayurvedic methods. The aim of treatment is to bring you back to your prakruti, where you can then follow the diet and lifestyle guidelines for your dosha type to maintain balance for lasting health and wellbeing.

Use the self-assessment chart on the following pages to determine your dosha type. Fill it out twice, using a tick for the prakruti, and a cross for the vikruti. For an objective view, you could also ask someone who knows you well to fill it out for you.

◀ VATA PEOPLE ARE LIGHT IN WEIGHT AND TALL OR VERY SHORT.

To determine your vikruti, concentrate upon your current condition and recent health history. To discover your prakruti, base your choices on what seems most consistently true over your whole lifetime. When you have finished, add up the marks under each dosha to discover your balance in prakruti and vikruti. Most people will have the highest score in one dosha. However, if your score is almost equal between two doshas, then you are probably a dual dosha type, or if equal between three, a tri-dosha type.

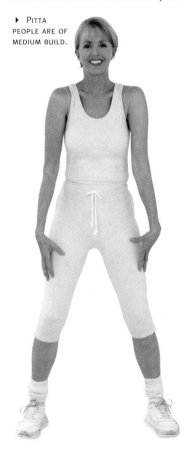

▶ PITTA PEOPLE ARE OF MEDIUM BUILD.

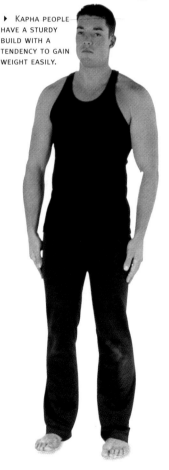

▶ KAPHA PEOPLE HAVE A STURDY BUILD WITH A TENDENCY TO GAIN WEIGHT EASILY.

which dosha are you?

	VATA	PITTA	KAPHA	V	P	K
Height	Tall or short and thin	Medium	Tall or short and sturdy	☐	☐	☐
Musculature	Thin, prominent tendons	Medium/firm	Plentiful/solid	☐	☐	☐
Bodily frame	Light, narrow	Medium	Large/broad	☐	☐	☐
Weight	Light, hard to gain	Medium	Heavy, gains easily	☐	☐	☐
Sweat	Minimal	Profuse, especially when hot	Moderate	☐	☐	☐
Skin	Dry, cold	Soft, warm	Moist, cool, possibly oily	☐	☐	☐
Complexion	Darkish	Fair/pink/ red/freckles	Pale/white	☐	☐	☐
Hair amount	Average	Early thinning and greying	Plentiful	☐	☐	☐
Type of hair	Dry/thin/ dark/coarse	Fine/soft/ red/fair	Thick, lustrous brown	☐	☐	☐
Size of eyes	Small, narrow or sunken	Average	Large, prominent	☐	☐	☐
Type of eyes	Dark brown or grey, dull	Blue/grey/ hazel, intense	Blue, brown, attractive	☐	☐	☐
Teeth and gums	Protruding, receding gums	Yellowish, gums bleed	White teeth, strong gums	☐	☐	☐
Size of teeth	Small or large, irregular	Average	Large	☐	☐	☐
Physical activity	Quick pace, active	Moderate, average	Slow, steady	☐	☐	☐
Endurance	Low	Good	Very good	☐	☐	☐
Strength	Poor	Good	Very good	☐	☐	☐

	VATA	PITTA	KAPHA	V	P	K
Temperature	Dislikes cold, likes warmth	Likes coolness	Aversion to cool and damp			
Digestion	Irregular, forms gas	Quick eating causes burning	Prolonged, forms mucus			
Stools	Tendency to constipation	Tendency to loose stools	Plentiful, slow elimination			
Lifestyle	Variable, erratic	Busy, tends to achieve a lot	Steady			
Sleep	Light, interrupted, fitful	Sound, short	Deep, likes plenty			
Emotional tendency	Fearful, anxious, insecure	Fiery, angry, judgemental	Greedy, possessive			
Mental activity	Restless, lots of ideas	Sharp, precise, logical	Calm, steady, stable			
Memory	Good recent memory	Sharp, generally good	Good long term			
Reaction to stress	Excites very easily	Quick temper	Not easily irritated			
Work	Creative	Intellectual	Caring			
Moods	Change quickly	Change slowly	Generally steady			
Speech	Fast	Clear, sharp, precise	Deep, slow			
Finances	Poor	Spends on luxuries	Rich, good at saving			
Resting pulse:						
Women	Above 80	70–80	Below 70			
Men	Above 70	60–70	Below 60			
			TOTALS			

vata types

Vata is the energy of movement, and regulates all activity in the body, both mental and physiological, including breathing, blinking and the beating of our hearts. All the impulses in the network of the nervous system are governed by vata.

Vata individuals usually have light, flexible bodies and tend not to gain weight easily. Their tendency is towards dry hair and cool skin and, with little fat to protect them, to feel the cold. Most vata types feel

▼ VATA IS A CREATIVE DOSHA – MANY ARTISTS, DANCERS AND WRITERS ARE VATA TYPES.

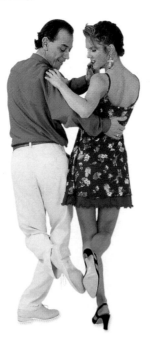

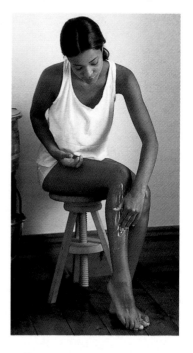

▲ VATA PEOPLE ARE PRONE TO EXCESSIVELY DRY SKIN, CRACKED HEELS AND DRY LIPS.

most comfortable during the spring and summer seasons.

Their constitution is delicate and their levels of energy erratic; they may find it hard to maintain order and structure in their daily lives, quickly becoming bored with routine or mundane tasks. A bundle of nervous energy, the vata type is always on the go, preferring to jog or work out rather than to sit down and take it easy. These individuals may find it hard to relax, which in turn can lead to insomnia and stress-related disorders.

Vata people are clear, quick thinkers, with a highly developed imaginative and intuitive faculty; some may possess clairvoyant abilities. Despite being fearful, anxious types, these people enjoy new challenges and love excitement: they seem to make major life changes, such as change of residence, partner, or employment for instance, much more frequently than other more "grounded" dosha types. This can easily upset their balance and lead to vata disorders.

BALANCED VATA CHARACTERISTICS

- flexible
- artistic, creative
- imaginative, inventive
- changeable
- fresh, light
- emotions: joy and happiness

EXCESS VATA SYMPTOMS

- digestive disorders: constipation, flatulence
- lower back pain, sciatica, arthritis
- nervous disorders
- premenstrual tension
- mental confusion, hyperactivity, restlessness
- emotions: fearful, nervous, anxious, capricious, impatient, irritable

▶ VATA PEOPLE ARE PRONE TO DRY HAIR.

GUIDELINES FOR BALANCING VATA

- keep warm
- slow down and stay calm
- eat regular meals
- eat cooked, rather than raw food
- spend time alone
- keep a regular routine
- put energy into creative pursuits

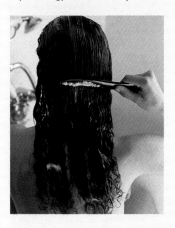

pitta types

Pitta is the energy of metabolism. It governs all the bio-chemical changes that take place in the body, regulating temperature and digestion, absorption and assimilation – not only of food, but also environmental, external stimuli.

Pittas have a strong constitution; they enjoy their food and have a healthy appetite. Their body type is usually of average build and nicely proportioned, seldom gaining or losing much weight. Generally they have straight, fine, fair hair and skin that is sensitive to the sun. Their eyes are bright and typically blue, greyish-green or coppery brown. Pittas tend to be

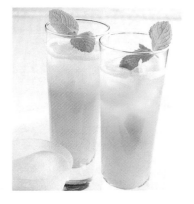

▲ PITTA TYPES MAY NEED TO DRINK MORE IN ORDER TO STAY COOL.

▼ TO BALANCE THEIR WORKAHOLIC NATURE PITTA PEOPLE SHOULD MAKE SURE THEY SPEND TIME IN NATURAL SURROUNDINGS.

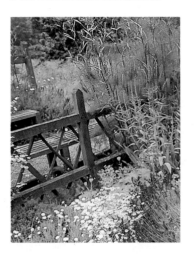

warm and sweat easily, and are aggravated by hot, humid weather.

Pitta types have a keen intel-lect and a logical, enquiring mind. They love planning and order, and make good leaders and public speakers; they are often attracted to professions such as medicine, engineering and the law, as they enjoy the challenge of going deeply into problems to find a solution. Ambitious, determined and aggres-sive by nature, their deep-seated fear of failure drives them to succeed. Pitta types are often found reading or working late into the night and many become workaholics, burning their energy through too much mental activity.

Their perfectionist tendencies can make them impatient and intolerant – both towards others and themselves – whereupon they become critical, impatient and judgemental. They are also quick to flare up in anger and are inclined towards jealousy.

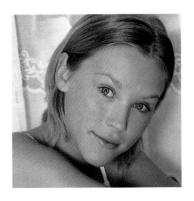

▲ Pitta people have a good sense of humour and a warm personality.

Balanced Pitta Characteristics

- keen intellect
- meticulous and precise
- capacity for leadership and organization
- enjoys new challenges
- emotions: happiness, humour, warmth

Excess Pitta Symptoms

- fevers
- diarrhoea
- inflammatory diseases
- acid indigestion
- skin rashes, eczema
- eye disorders
- premature greying, hair loss
- emotions: anger, hate, irritability, jealousy, envy, fear, bewilderment

▶ Pitta people benefit from cooling showers.

Guidelines for Balancing Pitta

- stay cool: cool showers, cool environments, cool drinks
- avoid hot, spicy food
- take time off to relax and slow down
- relax in natural surroundings
- drink more water

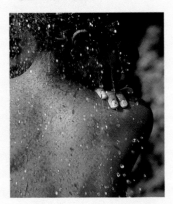

kapha types

This is the energy of stability, forming the body's structure and supplying the fluids that lubricate the joints, moisturize the skin and heal wounds. It creates and repairs the body's cells, maintains immunity and nourishes our emotions.

The kapha body type is well built, with strong muscles and large, heavy bones. Kapha individuals have thick or fine or wavy hair, smooth skin and large, attractive eyes. They enjoy deep, prolonged sleep and have a steady appetite and thirst, but their slow metabolism and digestion means they have a tendency to gain weight easily, especially if they don't take enough exercise. Although they are naturally athletic and have plenty of stamina, they are not easily motivated into action – a typical kapha type is happy to sit, eat and do nothing. Winter and early spring are the most difficult seasons for a kapha, when the weather is heavy, wet and cold and it is even more difficult to get motivated to keep exercising regularly.

The kapha individual dislikes change and is happiest following a

▼ KAPHA PEOPLE ARE LOVING AND DEPENDABLE BY NATURE.

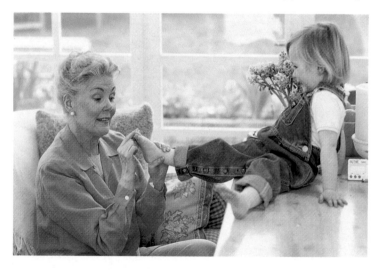

regular routine. They are steady, methodical, practical and pragmatic people – the workers who can be relied upon to get a job done. They have good organizational skills and usually make excellent managers. Additionally, their warm, loving, sensitive nature makes them well suited to the caring professions. Their calm, grounded presence instils confidence in others, acting as a steadying influence on those who are "all over the place".

It is easy for kapha people to get stuck in a rut and fall into lethargy and depression. Once depressed, it becomes even more difficult for them to motivate themselves, and they frequently turn to food for emotional support.

BALANCED KAPHA CHARACTERISTICS
- strength and stamina
- slow and steady
- health and vigour
- good long-term memory
- practical and reliable
- emotions: sweet, loving, sensitive, patient, nurturing

EXCESS KAPHA SYMPTOMS
- congestion
- excess mucus: bronchial/nasal discharge
- sluggish digestion
- slow mental responses
- obesity and fluid retention
- diabetes
- depression
- too much sleep
- emotions: stubbornness, greed, jealousy, possessiveness, lethargy

▶ KAPHA PEOPLE BENEFIT FROM REGULAR EXERCISE.

GUIDELINES FOR BALANCING KAPHA
- wear bright, strong and invigorating colours
- take regular exercise
- avoid heavy, sweet food and dairy products
- vary your routine
- keep active

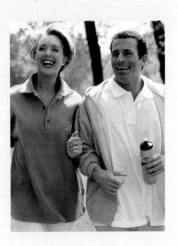

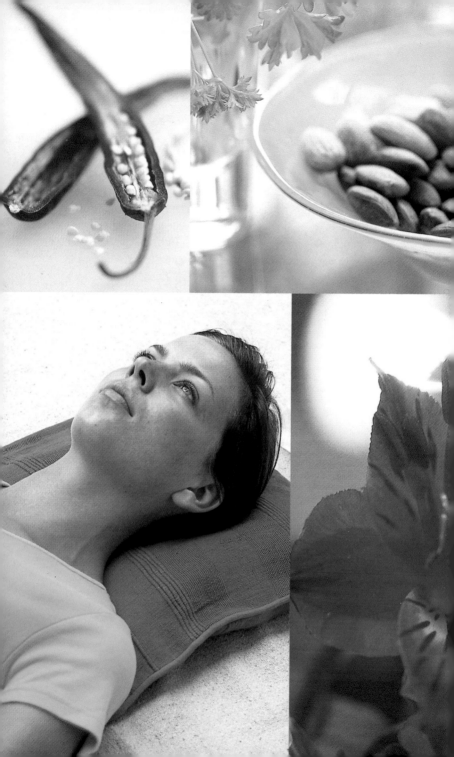

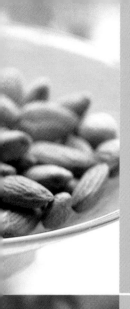

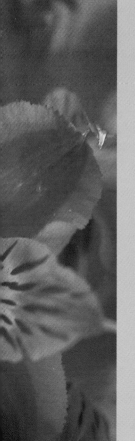

a formula for living

Ayurveda is a comprehensive healthcare system; it is interested in the whole person and all aspects of living. Having established your doshic constitution (prakruti) and any current imbalances (vikruti), Ayurveda gives extensive guidelines on how you can work with the doshas to maintain balance and harmony. At the root of all Ayurvedic treatment is diet; eating to suit the dominant dosha is the primary method used to prevent and treat disease. A healthy lifestyle is achieved through exercise, minimizing stress and by adjusting our behaviour to suit the natural rhythms of life, including the seasons and time of day. Ayurveda also draws upon a wide range of healing arts, including crystal and colour therapy, massage and essential oils, to purify and strengthen the body and balance the doshas.

vata dietary guidelines

Nourishing stews, warming soups and hot, spicy food are good for vata people, whereas cold, raw food is best avoided. To balance their restless nature, they should eat at regular times in a calm, relaxing atmosphere.

HERBS AND SPICES
best source: most of them – particularly warming or sweet herbs; asafoetida helps with the digestion of food.
avoid: caraway.

GRAINS
best source: cooked oats, quinoa, rice, and wheat.
avoid: barley, buckwheat, rye, corn, cereals (cold, dry or puffed), couscous, muesli (granola) and millet.

BEANS, PEAS AND LENTILS
best source: chickpeas, mung beans, red lentils.
avoid: all, except those listed.

MEAT, FISH AND EGGS
best source: beef, chicken, duck, freshwater or sea-fish, shellfish and turkey; boiled or scrambled eggs.
avoid: lamb, pork, rabbit and venison.
• Meat and fish are grounding and strengthening for vata.

▼ ALL TYPES OF NUTS AND SEEDS ARE GOOD FOR VATA IF EATEN IN MODERATION.

▼ ALL FRESH, RIPE FRUITS ARE GOOD FOR THE VATA DIET.

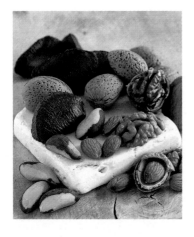

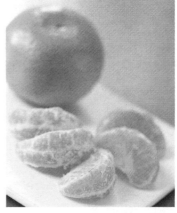

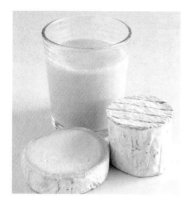

▲ DAIRY PRODUCTS ARE GOOD, ESPECIALLY COW'S AND GOAT'S MILK AND SOFT CHEESE.

VEGETABLES

best source: asparagus, beetroot (beet), carrots, courgettes (zucchini), cucumber, green beans, garlic, leeks, okra, olives, onions (cooked), parsnips, peas, pumpkins, spinach, swede (rutabaga), sweet potatoes and watercress.

avoid: beansprouts, broccoli, Brussels sprouts, cabbage, cauliflower; hot (bell) peppers, mushrooms and white potatoes.

• Cooked vegetables are better than those that are raw or dried.

FRUIT

best source: most ripe, sweet fruit.
avoid: cranberries, dried fruit, pears, persimmon, pomegranate, unripe fruit and watermelon.

COOKING OILS

best source: unrefined sesame oil.

SWEETENERS

best source: in moderation: honey, maple syrup and unrefined cane sugar products.
avoid: white sugar.

DRINKS

best source: some fruit juices, beer or wine in moderation, hot dairy drinks, herbal teas, especially chamomile, lavender, licorice, fresh ginger, peppermint and rosehip.
avoid: black tea, coffee, carbonated drinks, ice-cold drinks – tomato, cranberry, pear and apple juice.

▼ HOT CHOCOLATE IS A GOOD CHOICE OF HOT DRINK IF IT IS MADE WITH MILK.

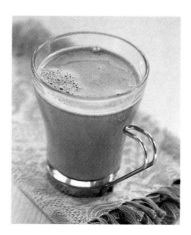

pitta dietary guidelines

Pitta people should choose foods that are cooling and soothing, and avoid hot, sour, spicy dishes and fatty, fried or oily food. It is important to eat when hungry, as pitta types easily suffer low blood-sugar levels and become irritable.

HERBS AND SPICES

best source: aloe vera juice (not to be used in pregnancy), basil leaves, cinnamon, coriander (cilantro), cumin, dill, fennel, fresh ginger, hijiki, mint leaves and spearmint.

avoid: all hot spices, cayenne and chilli peppers, garlic, salt, vinegar, mustard seeds and ketchup.

GRAINS

best source: barley, oats, wheat, and rice (especially white basmati).

avoid: brown rice, buckwheat, corn, millet and rye.

▼ CINNAMON IS A MILD, VERSATILE SPICE THAT IS A GOOD CHOICE FOR PITTA PEOPLE.

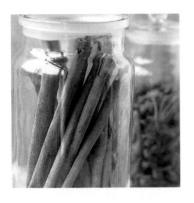

BEANS, PEAS AND LENTILS

best source: all beans, chickpeas, tofu and other unfermented soya products.

avoid: green lentils (except in soup) and red lentils; miso, soy sauce.

NUTS AND SEEDS

best source: almonds, coconut, pumpkin and sunflower seeds.

avoid: all others, particularly cashew nuts and sesame seeds.

MEAT, FISH AND EGGS

best source: in strict moderation: chicken, freshwater fish, rabbit, turkey and venison.

avoid: red meat, all seafood and egg yolk.

VEGETABLES

best source: most, especially asparagus, broccoli, green leaf vegetables, green lettuce, chicory.

avoid: carrots, aubergines (eggplant), spinach, radishes, onions, raw beetroot (beet), green olives, peppers, kohlrabi and tomatoes.

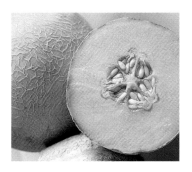

• Include plenty of salads and raw, rather than cooked vegetables in your diet.

FRUIT
best source: fully ripe, sweet, fresh fruit, including apples, apricots, avocados, berries, cherries, dates, figs, mangoes, melons, papaya, pears and plums.
avoid: citrus fruits, fruits with a sour or sharp, tangy taste such as cranberries, rhubarb, strawberries and green grapes.

DAIRY PRODUCTS
best source: most in moderation.
avoid: salted butter, buttermilk, sour cream and yogurt.

COOKING OILS
best source: in moderation: olive, sunflower, soya, coconut and walnut oils.
avoid: almond, corn and sesame oils.

SWEETENERS
best source: most in moderation.
avoid: honey and molasses.

DRINKS
best source: most sweet fruit juices, cow's milk, soya milk, rice milk mixed vegetable juice, beer and black tea.
avoid: hard spirits, wine, caffeinated drinks, sour or sharp fruit juices (such as berry juices), tomato juice and any ice-cold drinks.

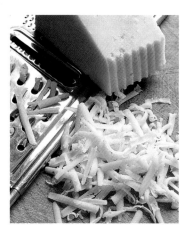

kapha dietary guidelines

Kapha food should be light, dry, hot and stimulating. Opt for cooked foods in preference to salads but go easy on rich sauces. Dairy products, sweet, sour and salty tastes and an excessive intake of wheat all aggravate kapha.

HERBS AND SPICES
best source: all pungent spices – ginger, black pepper, coriander (cilantro), turmeric and cardamon.
avoid: salt.

GRAINS
best source: barley, buckwheat, corn, couscous, millet, oat bran, polenta, rye.
avoid: oat flakes, pasta, wheat and rice (brown and white).

▼ MOST BEANS ARE GOOD FOR THE KAPHA DIET.

NUTS AND SEEDS
best source: pumpkin and sunflower seeds.
avoid: all nuts.

BEANS, PEAS AND LENTILS
avoid: kidney beans, soy beans (and their products), tofu (cold) and miso.

MEAT, FISH AND EGGS
best source: in strict moderation:

▼ FRESHWATER FISH IS BETTER THAN SEA-WATER FISH FOR KAPHAS.

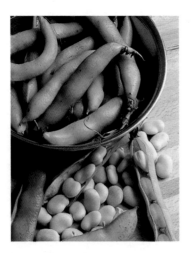

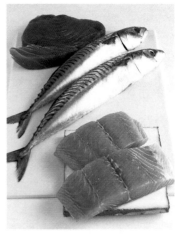

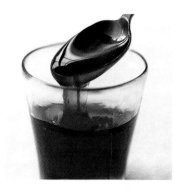

▲ Honey is the best sweetener, but you should avoid sugar and molasses.

scrambled eggs, poultry, prawns (shrimp), rabbit and venison.
avoid: beef, lamb, pork, seafood (except prawns/shrimp).

Vegetables
best source: most.
avoid: sweet vegetables, such as courgettes (zucchini), cucumber, parsnips, sweet potatoes, pumpkin, squash and tomatoes.
• Cooked vegetables are best.

Fruit
best source: apples, apricots, berries, cherries, cranberries, peaches, pears, pomegranates, prunes and raisins.
avoid: bananas, kiwi fruits, avocados, coconuts, dates, melons, olives, papaya, plums and pineapple.

• Sharp, astringent fruits are better than sweet or sour ones.

Cooking Oils
best source: corn, almond or sunflower oil.
• Use fats and oils sparingly.

Drinks
best source: fresh fruit and vegetable juices, black tea, herbal teas, hot soy milk drinks, dry red or white wine very occasionally.
avoid: fizzy, caffeinated drinks, coffee, orange juice, tomato juice and iced drinks.

▼ Squash is a sweet-tasting vegetable and should be avoided by kapha people. Sweet foods hinder a kapha's energy.

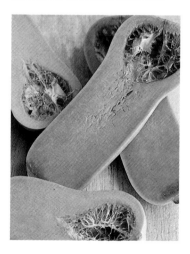

kapha dietary guidelines **31**

optimum living

Ayurveda stresses the importance of living a balanced life. It is all very well following the dietary guidelines for our dosha type, but if we neglect to take care of ourselves in the rest of our lives, then our efforts will be less effective.

Regular exercise plays an important role in staying healthy for all dosha types. It keeps the body strong and stimulates the digestive system to work more effectively.

Kaphas will get the most benefit from vigorous exercise, such as running, fast swimming, aerobics and fitness training, which will help to cleanse the body and dispel sluggish, lazy feelings. Kaphas should exercise more when the weather is cold and damp. Pittas require a moderate amount of

▼ THE TYPE OF EXERCISE YOU SHOULD DO IS DETERMINED BY YOUR CONSTITUTION.

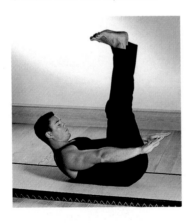

exercise, done for the fun of it rather than to be top dog; jogging, team sports and tai chi are all good. Vata people benefit from gentle, relaxing forms of exercise. They are the most easily exhausted of the dosha types, so they should not overdo things. Walking, yoga and slow swimming are ideal, although vata people can undertake most sports and activities, so long as they don't push themselves beyond their limits.

ROUTINE

Keeping a regular routine for vital activities such as sleeping, eating, exercising, bathing and working helps us to maintain balance in our lives. Ayurveda recommends harmonizing our internal body clock with the natural rhythm of the day. Long-distance travel, working night shifts, and eating at irregular times can all throw our body clock, and the doshas, off balance, making us feel out of sorts and out of harmony with those around us.

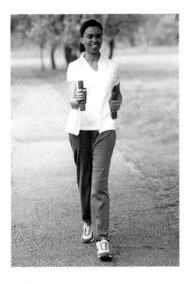

▲ WE ARE AT OUR MOST ACTIVE BETWEEN 10AM AND 2PM.

THE DAILY CYCLE

Ayurveda divides the day into two cycles, which roughly correspond with day and night. Each cycle has three phases, governed by one of the doshas.

DAY

06.00–10.00 kapha time of day. The body is gathering energy to begin the day. This is the best time for purification rituals (shower, cleansing, eliminating), yoga and meditation. Eat a light breakfast.

10.00–14.00 pitta time of day. The appetite is strongest at lunch-time so have your main meal of the day between these hours.

14.00–18.00 vata time of day. This is the most creative and communicative time of the day. Take a regular break to avoid activity turning into stress. The late afternoon is a good time to meditate.

NIGHT

18.00–22.00 kapha time of night. The body tires. Eat a light meal and take a walk to aid digestion.

22.00–02.00 pitta time of night. Avoid strenuous activity. Go to bed at a reasonable hour.

02.00–06.00 vata time of night. The body shuts down.

▼ ALL DOSHAS SHOULD ADOPT A ROUTINE THAT ADHERES TO THE NATURAL RHYTHM OF THE DAY AND NIGHT.

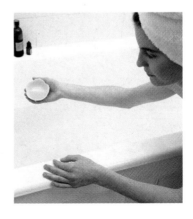

the cycles of life

The seasons of the year show us that life is cyclical; an everlasting round of gestation, birth, growth, decline and death. The doshas are inevitably related to these natural laws and follow this regenerative cycle.

The doshas are sensitive to changes in weather conditions, which loosely tie in with the seasons. Vata is highest in autumn and early winter, and at times of dry, cold and windy weather. The pitta season is late spring and summer and during times of heat and humidity. Kapha is highest in the winter months and during early spring when the weather is cold and damp.

Ayurveda recommends that we take these seasonal changes into account when we are planning our eating and lifestyle habits, as the weather can aggravate or cause doshic imbalance. For instance, during the cold, damp months of winter, kapha accumulates. This leads to more "damp" in the body in the form of excess mucus, and is the traditional season for coughs and colds. This is made much more likely if your diet is high in foods that aggravate the kapha condition – lots of dairy products and heavy, rich food – and more likely still if

▼ SPRING IS THE TIME TO CONSIDER A
CLEANSING FAST TO CLEAR EXCESS KAPHA.

▼ SUMMER IS THE SEASON OF HEAT.
COUNTER IT WITH SOOTHING ACTIVITIES.

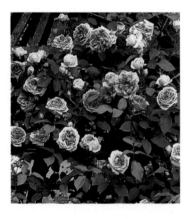

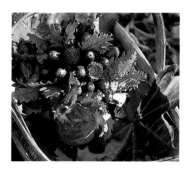

▲ Autumn is the season of changeable weather and increased levels of vata.

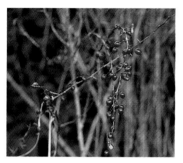

▲ Kapha people find it hard to motivate themselves in winter.

you are a kapha or have a kapha imbalance (vikruti).

If you are a dual or tri-dosha type, work with whichever dosha predominates at any given time. For example, if you are a vata-pitta type, choose foods from the pitta eating plan during the summer months and from the vata plan during the autumn and winter.

The Stages of Life

Ayurveda also sees the human life span in terms of the doshas.

0–30 years – kapha: this is the time of growth and development.

30–60 years – pitta: we apply the skills and knowledge of our kapha years to this time of life.

60+ years – vata: physical decline and spiritual growth.

WEATHER/SEASON	VATA	PITTA	KAPHA	BEST ACTION
warming up (spring)	neutral	accumulating	aggravated	cleansing fast to clear excess kapha
hot (summer)	accumulating	aggravated	decreasing	wear cooling colours, eat raw foods, rest and relax
cooling (autumn)	aggravated	decreasing	neutral	stay warm and comfortable; follow a regular routine
cold (winter)	decreasing	neutral	accumulating	treat kapha dosha with spices and warm drinks

yoga

An important element of Ayurvedic therapy is yoga as an exercise and a therapy. It is not only a physical discipline that helps to keep the body strong and supple, but it also calms the mind and helps us to find inner peace.

Yoga works with a variety of techniques, including physical postures, breathing exercises, relaxation and meditation. In its purest form it is a preparation for spiritual enlightenment, but it is also an effective therapy in the treatment of stress and chronic disease conditions.

Vata types are particularly suited to the gentle, rhythmic nature of yoga exercise, but all three doshas can benefit from yoga.

STANDING WARM-UPS

Before practising yoga, it is best to warm-up and stretch out the body. Stand relaxed but tall with the spine erect and the feet hip-width apart. Bring your hands together in front of your chest into prayer position. Raise your arms to the sides and come up on to your toes. Breathe in and stretch the arms up. Then breathe out to lower the arms and heels. Get a vigorous swinging movement going, opening the chest, stretching the spine and "waking up" the circulation.

SALUTE TO THE SUN

The following routine is best practised on rising first thing in the morning. The sequence should be repeated between two and six times. It is a good exercise to get yourself moving and release sluggish, tired feelings.

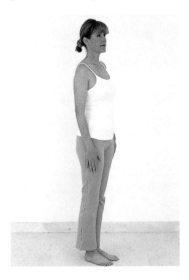

1 Stand upright with your hands at your side, knees and shoulders relaxed and your neck fully extended upwards. Inhale.

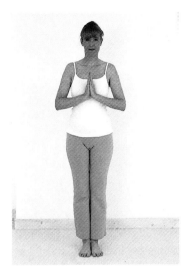

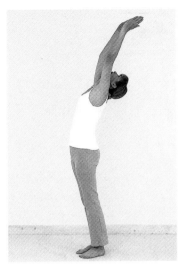

2 Look straight ahead. Breathe out while bringing the palms of your hands together at chest height into the prayer position.

3 Breathe in deeply. Keeping your hands together, raise your hands over your head. Arch your back as far as is comfortable. Exhale slowly.

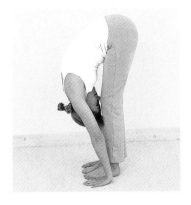

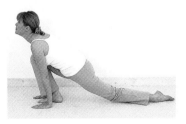

4 Bend forward to touch the floor if you can, at each side of your feet.

5 Breathing in, bend your right knee and slide and extend your left leg out behind you. Your knee rests on the floor. Put the hands on the floor. Extend your neck upwards. ▶

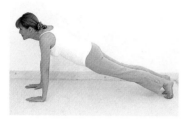
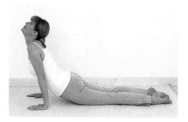

6 With your hands flat on the floor, extend your right leg out to meet your left leg. Take your weight up on to your hands and your toes. Keep the neck straight. Breathe out. Lower the body flat to the ground.

7 Supporting the weight of your upper body on your arms, raise your chest, stomach and pelvic bones from the ground. Extend your neck upwards. Exhale slowly. Breathing in, lower your stomach and pelvis back down to the floor.

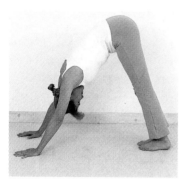

8 In one movement, raise your bottom and pull yourself up into an arch. Extend your arms and legs fully. Lower your heels towards the floor (but don't strain). Bend the left knee so that it touches the ground part way between your right foot and hands. Bring the right foot to the side of the left knee.

TYPES OF YOGA

There are many different types of yoga. The most widely practised in the West is "Hatha" yoga. Hatha yoga is just one branch of yoga and within this branch there are various sub-categories.

• Astanga Vinyasa: a fast series of challenging postures performed using synchronized breathing. This is probably the most aerobic form of yoga.

• Iyengar: alignment and precision of movement are used to enhance posture, breathing and flexibility.

• Kundalini: breathing techniques and prana (life force) are worked on to balance the body's energy and achieve relaxation.

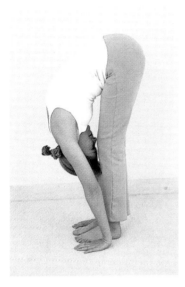

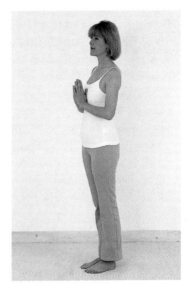

9 Move your hands back to your feet and return to position 4

10 Breathe in deeply as you raise your torso and repeat step 2.

 11 Breathe out slowly as you lower your arms and return to the starting position. Look straight ahead, allow your breathing to return to normal, then repeat the whole sequence with the other leg.

Caution

This sequence is not suitable during pregnancy, the menstrual cycle, if you are suffering from any physical injury, or back pain.

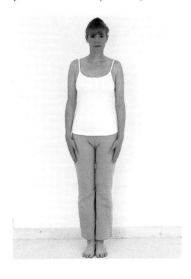

yoga breathing

Yoga teaches special breathing techniques as an aid to relaxation and meditation. Alternate nostril breathing has a calming effect on the nervous system and a balancing influence. It is best done after yoga and before meditation.

Sit upright in a comfortable position, either on a chair or cross-legged on the floor with your back straight. Make sure the chest and abdomen are not restricted by tight clothing. Close your eyes, empty your mind and breathe deeply in and out a few times in a relaxed way.

CAUTION
Do not restrict the breathing or hold your breath. Instead concentrate on breathing in with deep breaths, then exhaling slowly. If you start to feel dizzy, rest for a moment, open your eyes and breathe normally. Resume when you feel comfortable.

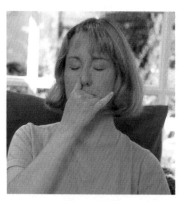

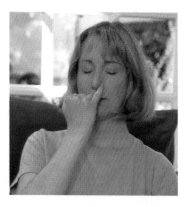

1 Bring your right hand in front of your face, with the three middle fingers tucked in towards your palm and the thumb and little finger extended. Place your thumb on your right nostril to close it, and breathe in through your left nostril.

2 Close the left nostril with your little finger. Breathe out through the right nostril. Holding the hand in position, breathe in through the right nostril. Close it with your thumb, open the left nostril by lifting your finger and breathe out.

deep relaxation

Relaxation is an essential part of yoga practise. During relaxation the mind and body unwind and deep-seated tensions dissolve away. The classic yoga pose for relaxation is called the corpse pose. Do this exercise at any time.

Lie on your back with your feet apart and your arms slightly away from your sides. Roll the feet and hips in and out to find the best position, then roll the hands and shoulders in and out. If your chin juts up, place a small cushion under your head. If your waist arches, place a cushion under your knees. It takes time to find a relaxing position, but it's well worth it.

When you are comfortable, allow your breathing to settle and then slow it down, feeling your body soften, as if you are melting into the floor. Relax in this position for several minutes. To come out of the pose, stretch your arms and legs and slowly open your eyes. You should feel refreshed.

CAUTION

Do not lie flat on your back if you are more than 30 weeks pregnant or have breathing problems. Recline instead, with your back supported by cushions or a beanbag.

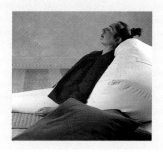

▼ LET YOUR MIND EMPTY OF THOUGHTS, OTHERWISE YOU WILL NOT BENEFIT FROM THIS EXERCISE. ONCE YOU HAVE FOUND A COMFORTABLE POSITION, VISUALIZE YOURSELF COLLECTING YOUR THOUGHTS TOGETHER, CARRYING THEM OUT OF THE ROOM AND LEAVING THEM OUT THERE.

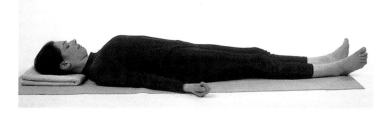

relaxing meditation

Meditation is food for the soul. Its effect is to deep-clean the mind and transform the emotions, leaving us feeling refreshed and calm. It is one of the most important methods in Ayurveda for permanently stabilizing the doshas.

Ayurvedic practitioners believe that toxins (ama) in the body also have their emotional and mental counterparts. Emotional states, such as greed, envy, jealousy and anger, negative thoughts and compulsive behaviour patterns create psychic "dirt" or emotional ama. They are as detrimental to our health as the chemical stress hormones produced by the body.

DAILY MEDITATION

Make meditation a part of your daily routine. Practise it for 10–15 minutes a day. Sunrise and sunset are the best times to meditate, but find a time that is convenient for you and stick to it. Some people like to use a (gentle) alarm to indicate when the session is finished.

1 Find a quiet place where you won't be disturbed. Either sit on a straight-backed chair or cross-legged on the floor. It is important that you are relaxed and comfortable and that your spine is straight.

2 Place your hands, palms upmost, on your thighs. Alternatively, rest your hands on your knees or on a small cushion on your lap.

3 Close your eyes and become aware of your breathing. With every out-breath, think "letting go".

4 Focus your attention inwards, allowing any noises or distractions outside to fade away.

▼ THE CLASSIC YOGA POSE, THE LOTUS POSITION, HAS BECOME SYMBOLIC OF RELAXATION AND MEDITATION. HOWEVER, IT TAKES SUPPLE JOINTS AND PRACTISE TO ACHIEVE IT.

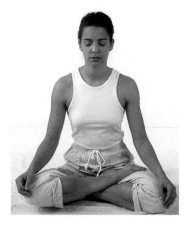

5 Don't try to control your mind – either by trying to hold on to a particular thought, or by rejecting any other. Meditation is about accepting what you find and allowing it to be there. Just allow your mind to wander.

6 Remember to stay focused on your breath (this will naturally help to quieten the mind) and keep your body relaxed.

7 When you are ready, open your eyes and let yourself return to normal waking consciousness. Slowly get up and have a good stretch, ready to face the world again with renewed vigour.

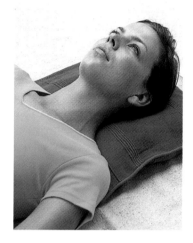

▲ YOU CAN MEDITATE LYING DOWN, BUT DON'T CHOOSE A BED FOR YOUR SURFACE OR YOU MAY FIND YOURSELF FALLING ASLEEP.

▼ AT THE END OF YOUR MEDITATION, HUG YOUR KNEES INTO YOUR CHEST, THEN STRETCH OUT YOUR LIMBS.

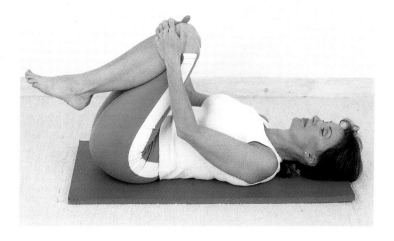

relaxing meditation **43**

the radiance of colour

Colour is a delight to our visual sense and its subtle vibrations affect us on all levels of our being. Ayurvedic treatments make use of the healing powers of colour to restore or stabilize the balance between the three doshas.

COLOURS AND THE DOSHAS

We can use colour to influence our wellbeing in the clothes we wear, the food we eat, and in our environment. The vibrations of certain colours help or aggravate each of the doshas.

VATA

Energetic vata individuals benefit from most of the pastel colours and earthy colours that are gentle and warm to look at, such as ochres, browns and yellows. Brown and ochre help to draw energy down through the body's system, stabilizing and grounding the vata personality; yellow is linked to the mind and will help to keep the vata mentally alert. Minimize the use of dark and cool colours, such as blues, browns and black.

PITTA

Excess pitta (such as irritability and impatience) is balanced by wearing cooling and calming colours, such as green, blue, violet, or any quiet pastel shade. Blue is a healing colour and helps the pitta type to remain open without being over-stimulated; green soothes the emotions and encourages harmonious feelings; and violet increases awareness of spiritual issues. Reds and oranges can inflame the pitta dosha, and yellow, gold and black should be minimized.

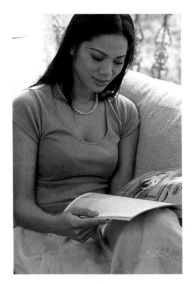

◀ PASTEL COLOURS ARE LIBERATING FOR VATA PEOPLE.

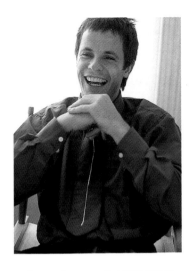

SOOTHING BLUE CALMS A PITTA PERSON.

KAPHA

The lethargy of kapha is balanced by bright, lively, bold colours, especially reds, oranges and warm pinks. Both reds and pinks are energizing and positive but red should be used sparingly as it may be over-stimulating. Orange is a warming, nourishing colour that feeds the sexual organs and helps to remove congestion in the system. Yellow and gold are also good colours for kapha, but greens, dark blues or white are best avoided.

KAPHA PEOPLE SHOULD CHOOSE VIBRANT COLOURS TO HELP MOTIVATE THEMSELVES INTO ACTION.

COLOUR INFUSIONS

In Ayurveda colour is an important healing tool. Different colours carry specific energies. To make a colour infusion wrap a piece of coloured fabric or film around a glass of water and leave it to stand in the sun for 4 hours. The water will become infused with the vibrations of that colour, and drinking it is said to bring beneficial results.

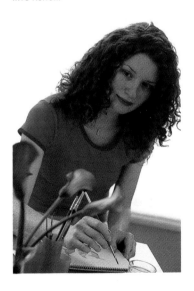

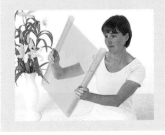

crystals & gems

All substances in nature are believed to contain the creative intelligence of the cosmos. Gems and crystals have healing energies that enliven the vital energy centres (chakras) in the body, and can be utilized to harmonize the doshas.

Stones are able to act as energy transmitters, having the power to store, magnify and transform energy. This means it is important to always clean any stone before it is used for healing purposes; leave it to soak in salt water overnight and then rinse thoroughly. Once the stone is free from any psychic "dirt", you can then make an infusion by placing it in a glass bowl of spring water and leaving it in sunlight for about 4 hours. Drain off the water and drink it.

Vata

Rose quartz balances excess vata and brings relief to conditions such as nervousness, dry skin and hair, constipation and bloating. Topaz is a warm stone that dispels fear and is ideal for calming vata anxiety; wear it when you want to feel confident and in control. Amethyst has balancing properties and is useful for troublesome emotional states or when clarity of mind is needed.

▼ CRYSTALS ARE IMPORTANT HEALING TOOLS IN AYURVEDA.

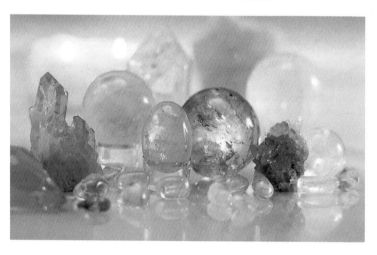

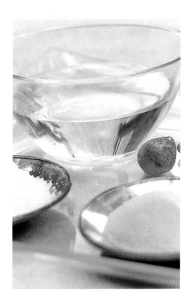

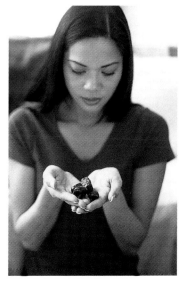

▲ Cleanse crystals in a bowl of salt water before use.

▲ Attune your attention to crystals to benefit from their energy.

It also helps to promote feelings of inner peace and harmony. Quartz crystal also helps to calm vata and enhances intuition.

Pitta

Pearls (or mother-of-pearl), red coral and moonstone are all good for reducing excess pitta. All three stones have a soft and cooling energy vibration that can help to calm inflammatory conditions, such as angry emotions, skin rashes, all "-itises", and acid indigestion. Amethyst encourages compassion and dignity and is also good for pitta imbalances.

Kapha

Deep red stones, such as ruby or garnet, stimulate kapha energy and balance the effects of excess kapha conditions, including water retention, lethargy, depression, weight problems and sinus and respiratory disorders. The refined, subtle vibrations of lapis lazuli will also help to lift excess kapha from its slow, heavy nature to something more light and ethereal.

aromas & massage

Our sense of smell is directly related to the balance of the doshas. Fragrant essential oils, extracted from hundreds of different plants and their components, can be used to balance the mind and heal the emotions.

Essential oils are inhaled and/or massaged into the skin. They should not be put directly on the skin or taken internally; some oils are contra-indicated in pregnancy or for some medical conditions.

Aromas and the Doshas

Warm, sweet, calming and earthy aromas balance vata. These include camphor, eucalyptus, ginger, musk, sandalwood and jatamansi (a spikenard species from India). A blend of basil, orange, geranium, and cloves is good for harmonizing vata imbalance, and other useful fragrances include lavender, pine and frankincense.

Pitta is soothed by cooling, calming, sweet aromas such as honeysuckle, jasmine, sandalwood and rose. Rose geranium, lemongrass, fennel or mint are helpful.

Warm and stimulating or spicy, earthy fragrances are helpful for kapha. These include eucalyptus, cinnamon, myrrh, thyme, basil, musk, camphor, cloves, rosemary, ginger and sage. Juniper oil is especially useful for lymphatic drainage.

▼ LOOKING AT A ROSE AS WELL AS SMELLING ONE LIFTS THE SPIRITS AND PROMOTES FEELINGS OF WELLBEING.

▼ ESSENTIAL OILS ARE APPLIED TO THE SKIN IN A "CARRIER" OIL, SUCH AS ALMOND OR WHEATGERM.

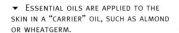

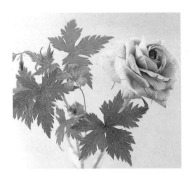

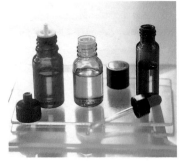

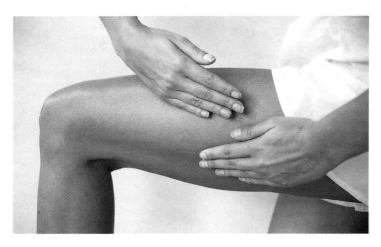

Massage and the Doshas

To massage with essential oils, add 7–10 drops of the chosen essential oil to 25ml/1½ tbsp carrier oil.

Vatas enjoy gentle, soothing and relaxing massage. Use stroking movements and pay attention to areas of tight, dry skin. Pitta massage should be calming and relaxing. Use deep and varied movements and go easy wherever there is stiffness or soreness.

A vigorous massage stimulates the sluggish kapha metabolism. Use fast and strong movements, using very little oil or none at all (talcum powder may be used instead). To encourage lymphatic drainage, pay particular attention to the hip and groin area and around the armpits.

▲ PITTAS SHOULD HAVE A SLOW MASSAGE RHYTHM AND AVOID SUDDEN MOVEMENTS.

▼ A DAILY FOOT AND HAND MASSAGE WILL ACT AS A GROUNDING AND STABILIZING INFLUENCE FOR VATAS.

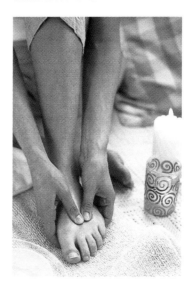

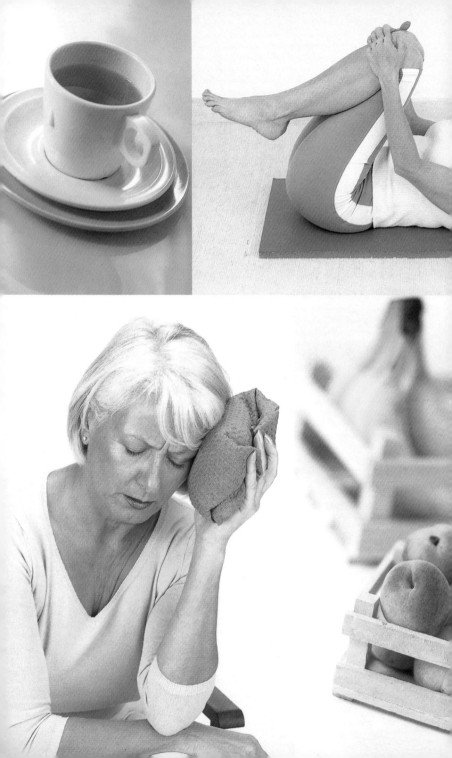

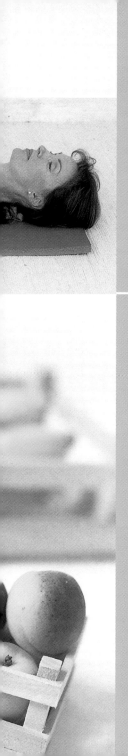

ayurveda for common ailments

In Ayurveda, health problems are treated according to the pattern of body type, or dosha. Some conditions may be vata, pitta or kapha, according to the symptoms, while others are generally linked with one dosha. Diarrhoea, for example, is a pitta condition, and constipation a vata one. When treating yourself you will need to discover whether your condition is displaying vata, pitta or kapha symptoms, and then follow the appropriate eating and lifestyle plan for that dosha to bring it back into balance. The treatments also recommend herbs and special Ayurvedic herbal mixtures, and offer tips on how to stay healthy. These herbs are available from Ayurveda suppliers and through the internet. Be sensible with your self-help regime and always consult a qualified Ayurvedic or medical doctor if your condition fails to respond to treatment.

digestive disorders

The gastro-intestinal tract is the most important part of the body, and the seat of the doshas. Our dosha type and lifestyle factors all influence the digestive system and each dosha is subject to particular disorders.

Regular bowel movements are a sign of a healthy gastro-intestinal tract (GI). Vata types are prone to irregular digestion and typical vata conditions include constipation, gas/flatulence, and tension (causing stomach cramps or spasms).

CONSTIPATION
Drinking a glass of hot water each morning will help to get things moving. Herbs include triphala and satisabgol (psyllium husks). Triphala is a special Ayurvedic combination of three herbal fruits. It should not

▼ BUY AYURVEDIC HERBS FROM A SPECIALIST STOCKIST.

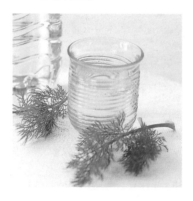

be used during pregnancy or if you suffer from ulcers of the GI. Satisabgol is gentle and soothing and a good "bulking" agent.

GAS, BLOATING, COLIC
If undigested food stays in the system for too long it begins to ferment, causing a range of unpleasant symptoms. Ayurvedic medicine recommends hingvastak, a herbal mix that includes asafoetida, ginger, black pepper and cumin.

Pitta digestion tends to be too fast. These types easily "burn" up food in anger or frustration and typical pitta problems include acidity and heartburn and diarrhoea.

ACIDITY AND HEARTBURN
Sip aloe vera juice to cool an inflamed digestive system (but not if you are pregnant). Use herbal preparations of shatavari, licorice (not to be used with high blood pressure or oedema) and amalki to balance acidity.

Diarrhoea

Avoid hot spices and eat small meals. Drink nettle tea to balance the digestive system and add coriander (cilantro), saffron, fresh ginger and nutmeg to your diet. A simple diet of rice, split mung dhal and vegetables is recommended while symptoms last.

The kapha metabolism is slow and problems of the GI lead to obesity, nausea, a build-up of mucus and poor circulation. Herbs for kapha conditions include trikatu ("three hot things"), which contains ginger, pippali and black pepper. Hot spices in general, such as chilli peppers, garlic and ginger are helpful for invigorating and cleansing the system. Regular vigorous exercise will help to keep kapha people moving and avoid stagnation.

◀ IF YOU HAVE A STOMACH UPSET, TRY TAKING A TONIC OF NETTLE TEA. IT WILL HELP TO BALANCE THE DIGESTIVE SYSTEM AND ALLEVIATE PITTA CONDITIONS.

▼ HERBAL TEAS ARE POWERFUL TONICS THAT ARE USED IN AYURVEDA.

▼ CHILLIES ARE GOOD FOR THE KAPHA DIET: THE HEAT OFFSETS THE SLUGGISH NATURE.

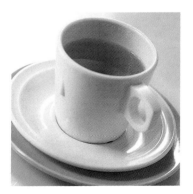

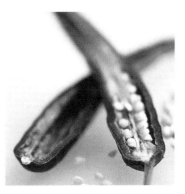

high blood pressure

Hypertension or high blood pressure is a potentially life-threatening condition and must be treated by a qualified medical practitioner. Ayurveda recommends steps that you can take which can help to bring it under control.

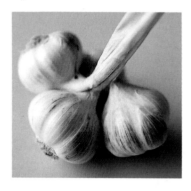

▲ EAT PLENTY OF GARLIC (RAW, FRESH IS BEST) AND TAKE REGULAR EXERCISE.

Lifestyle and diet play an important role in the prevention and treatment of hypertension. Physical and emotional stress cause the blood vessels to constrict and blood pressure to rise. Regular meditation and gentle yoga will help to counter this. A profound and simple way to relax is to lie in corpse pose for 10–15 minutes a day. Inverted postures (such as a headstand or a shoulderstand) and forward bending movements should be avoided.

Hypertension is often linked with high levels of cholesterol – increased lipids (fats) in the blood and fatty deposits on the artery walls, causing them to narrow. Stick to a kapha-reducing diet: avoiding dairy foods, especially hard cheeses, full-fat milk and sweet foods, salt, fried or cold food, cold drinks and red meat.

HONEY WATER

Add 5ml/1 tsp honey and 5–10 drops of apple cider vinegar or lime juice to a cup of hot water and drink a cup each morning. This helps to "scrape" fat from the system and lower cholesterol levels.

▼ LIMES ARE ACIDIC IN NATURE AND CAN HELP TO REDUCE CHOLESTEROL.

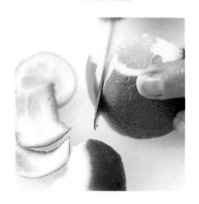

emotional stress

Our health is a complex interplay between our mind and emotions and our physical body. Mental and emotional stress can lead to physical ill-health and vice versa. Each of the doshas is prone to particular negative emotional states.

VATA

Of all the doshas, vata is the most prone to suffer the effects of stress. Anxiety, fear, insecurity, nervousness, restlessness and confusion are associated with increased vata. Slow down, eat regular, healthy meals and meditate each day. Fresh ginger and lemon tea are good tonics. A lavender, chamomile or jasmine oil massage is calming.

PITTA

Anger, criticism, irritability, frustration, envy and hostility are all signs of aggravated pitta. To cool the temper eat plain foods and cool drinks; avoid tea, coffee and alcohol. Focus on your emotions when you meditate. Include the following herbs in your diet: chamomile, coriander (cilantro), cumin, fennel, tulsi and sandalwood.

KAPHA

Boredom and a "can't be bothered" feeling are signs of unbalanced kapha. This dosha is associated with greed, possessiveness and attachment, which leads to overeating and to be "greedy" and smothering in relationships. Work with the kapha eating plan, and be sure to take plenty of vigorous exercise. Give the other more "space" in your relationships.

▼ A SOOTHING MASSAGE WON'T TAKE AWAY THE CAUSE OF YOUR EMOTIONAL STRESS BUT WILL HELP TO RELAX YOUR MIND AND BODY.

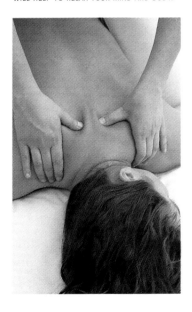

premenstrual syndrome

Every month, many women experience unpleasant physical and emotional symptoms 7–10 days before their period. For some it is severely debilitating. Ayurveda classifies the symptoms of premenstrual syndrome according to dosha type.

Lower-back pain, lower abdominal pain and bloating, coupled with anxiety, fearfulness, insomnia and marked mood swings are associated with vata imbalance. Take 15ml/1 tbsp aloe vera gel mixed with a pinch of black pepper three times a day before meals. Include the following herbs in your diet: dashamula, kaishore guggulu or yogaraj guggulu.

Pitta-type symptoms include irritability, tender breasts, hives, raised body temperature (hot flushes, sweats) and cystitis. Make a herbal mix of two parts shatavari to one part each of brahmi and musta. Take 2.5ml/½ tsp with warm water, twice a day. Alternatively, add a pinch of cumin powder to 15ml/ 1 tbsp aloe vera gel and take three times daily.

One of the main features of kapha premenstrual syndrome (PMS) is water retention; the breasts become heavy and swollen, and the legs, feet and ankles may also swell. Emotionally, the woman feels weepy, depressed and lethargic. Add a pinch of trikatu to 15ml/ 1 tbsp of aloe vera gel and take three times daily. Other herbs to include in your diet are purnarnava, kutki and musta.

◀ For many women PMS can be extremely debilitating. Make a record of your symptoms and do not ignore them.

Treatment Tips
To treat vata and kapha PMS, eat ten cherries a day on an empty stomach a week or so before the period starts.

low libido

Ayurveda acknowledges the importance of a healthy, ful-filling sex life. Our sex drive is affected by high stress levels, emotional factors and also by weakness or debility in the male or female reproductive organs.

Ayurveda suggests many foods that can strengthen the reproductive system. The following are equally suitable for both sexes.

Almonds
Soak ten almonds overnight. Peel them and eat before breakfast each day. Alternatively use them to make an almond milk drink. Blend them with a glass of warm milk, 5ml/ 1 tsp fructose, a pinch of nutmeg and a pinch of saffron.

Dates
Soak ten dates in ghee (a special form of clarified butter) with 1.5ml/¼ tsp of cardamon and a pinch of saffron. Cover and leave in a warm place for 2 weeks. Eat one date a day each morning; they taste delicious and will help with sexual debility and chronic fatigue.

Onions and Ginger
Take 15ml/1 tbsp onion juice with 5ml/1 tsp of fresh ginger juice twice a day.

Garlic Milk
Mix 250ml/8fl oz/1 cup milk, 50ml/ 2fl oz/¼ cup water and 1 chopped garlic clove. Boil to reduce the mixture. Drink at bedtime.

Herbal Treatments
Ayurvedic herbs to combat low libido include shatavari, ashwagandha, vidari, nutmeg and tagar.
For men Mix 5ml/1 tsp ashwagandha and 2.5ml/½ tsp vidari in a cup of warm milk and drink just before bedtime.
For women Substitute the ashwagandha with shatavari.

▼ Try eating three figs with 5ml/1 tsp of honey after breakfast.

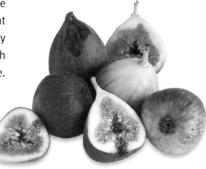

headaches

This common problem occurs for many reasons; headaches may be stress related, caused by diet or be related to infections, poor eyesight or bad posture. Ayurveda classifies headaches into vata, pitta and kapha type.

Throbbing vata-type headaches are caused by tension and anxiety. Ease muscle tension by massaging the neck and shoulders with sesame oil; rubbing sesame oil on the top of the head and on the soles of the feet at bedtime is also said to control vata. Ayurvedic herbs to include in your diet are triphala to clear any congestion, jatamansi, brahmi and calamus.

Pitta headaches are associated with heat or burning sensations, flushed skin and visual sensitivity to light. They can be brought on by eating spicy food and by anger or frustration. A pitta headache may clear up if you eat something sweet; try some fruit. Cooling aloe vera juice can help: take 30ml/ 2 tbsp up to three times a day.

Kapha headaches are congested, dull and heavy, and often associated with sinus pain. Fresh air and plenty of exercise will help to alleviate congestion.

▼ IF YOU HAVE A HEADACHE, YOUR BLOOD SUGAR MAY BE LOW. COUNTER THIS BY EATING SOMETHING SWEET – SUCH AS A PIECE OF FRUIT, RATHER THAN SUGARY TREATS.

▼ IF YOU SUFFER FROM FREQUENT HEADACHES, YOUR DIET MAY BE THE CAUSE OF YOUR DISCOMFORT. KEEP A RECORD TO SEE IF ANY FOODS TRIGGER YOUR HEADACHES.

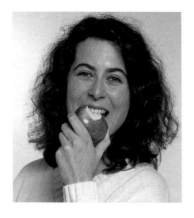

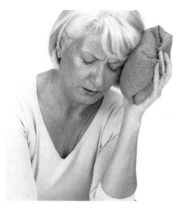

insomnia

People in the West are likely to have a problem with excess vata as it relates to overactivity in the nervous system and leads to stress-related disorders. Insomnia is caused by an increase of vata in the mind.

Any vata-increasing influence can contribute to insomnia, including lots of travel, stress, an erratic lifestyle and the use of stimulants such as tea or coffee. Ayurvedic herbal treatment is with brahmi, jatamansi, ashwagandha and nutmeg. A foot massage with brahmi oil last thing at night may help.

Out-of-balance pitta can also contribute to insomnia when it is brought on by anger, jealousy, frustration, fever, or excess sun or heat. Herbs to include in your diet are

▼ Tea, coffee, chocolate and cola contain caffeine, which keeps you awake.

brahmi, jatamansi, bhringaraj, shatavari and aloe vera juice. Massage brahmi oil into the head and feet.

INSOMNIA TREATMENT
As an aid to a good night's sleep, add 10ml/2 tsp fruit sugar and 2 pinches of grated nutmeg to a glass of tomato juice. Drink it late in the afternoon (16.00–17.00 hours) and follow it with an early dinner (18.00–19.00 hours).

▼ Spend time relaxing before you prepare for bed. You could scent the room with soothing essential oils.

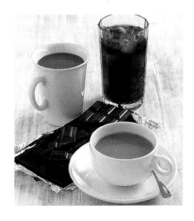

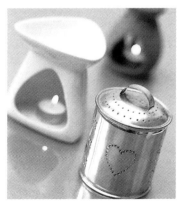

colds & flu

The cold damp months of winter and early spring are the times of year when many people will get a cold. Symptoms typically include excess mucus production and feverishness, alternately feeling chilly or burning hot.

Kapha colds are thick and mucous, with a heavy feeling in the head and/or body. Follow the kapha-eating plan and eliminate dairy, nuts and heavy, oily food from the diet. Drink hot lemon spiced with ginger, cinnamon and cloves or cardamon, and use steam inhalations to help clear the sinuses.

The early stage of a cold is often marked by a dry, sore throat. Dryness in the body is a symptom of vata imbalance; helpful herbs include ginger, cumin, pippali, tulsi, cloves, peppermint, shatavari and ashwagandha.

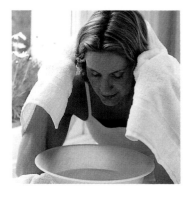

▲ A STEAM INHALATION, MADE USING GINGER ADDED TO A BOWL OF HOT WATER, HELPS RELIEVE A COLD.

When there is fever, a pitta imbalance may be indicated. Avoid hot, spicy food and use cooling herbal preparations; peppermint, spearmint, sandalwood, chrysanthemum and tulsi are all suitable.

GINGER
The best remedy for colds is ginger. It can be eaten raw, steeped in hot water and made into drinks. Its warming properties will invigorate the body and help with the elimination of toxins.

▼ MOST PEOPLE GET COLDS IN WINTER DURING THE KAPHA PHASE OF THE YEAR.

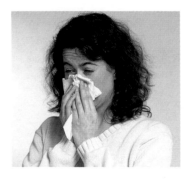

coughs

Coughs are usually a by-product of colds and other respiratory infections. They fall into two broad categories: those that are dry and irritating, and those that are "wet" and congesting. Inflammation may be present in either type.

Vata coughs are dry and irritating with very little mucus. They may be accompanied by a dry mouth and sore throat. Herbs and spices include licorice (contra-indicated if you suffer hypertension), shatavari, ashwagandha and cardamon. A ripe banana mashed up with 5ml/1 tsp of honey and a couple of pinches of black pepper is also effective; eat it two or three times a day.

Pitta coughs are usually associated with a lot of phlegm, which tends to stick on the chest. Fever or heat, combined with a burning sensation in the chest or throat may also be present. The best herbs for pitta coughs include peppermint, tulsi and sandalwood.

Kapha coughs are generally loose and productive. Keep warm and avoid damp, cold environments. A simple and effective treatment is to mix 2.5ml/½ tsp of black pepper with 5ml/1 tsp of honey and eat it on a full stomach. The heat of the black pepper will warm the body and help to drive out the cough. Ginger, lemons and cloves are also useful.

▼ TREAT A COUGH ACCORDING TO YOUR DOSHA TYPE.

▼ MAKE A WARMING LEMON DRINK TO SOOTHE A DRY COUGH.

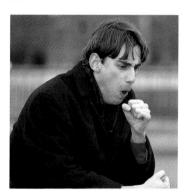

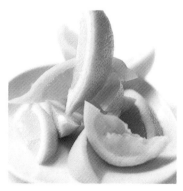

skin problems

A glowing complexion and silky, "baby-soft" skin is a reality that many of us only dream about. Skin problems are extremely common and can range in severity from the occasional spot to chronic conditions such as psoriasis.

Vata skin problems will be dry and rough and include chapped lips, cracked heels, "sandpaper" hands and dandruff. Avoid letting the skin dry out and exposing it to cold and/or windy weather. Herbal remedies for vata skin are triphala and satisabgol (the latter is useful if you are also constipated).

Excess pitta causes skin problems that itch, burn or erupt into spots or rashes. The skin is usually red, swollen, raised or inflamed, often with a yellow head or pus discharge. Avoid sun, heat, hot baths or saunas, and increase your

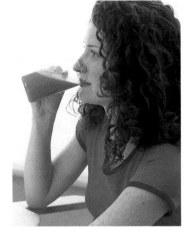

▲ JUICES ARE GOOD FOR THE SKIN. DRINK THEM WHEN THEY ARE FRESHLY MADE.

intake of water, salads, raw vegetables and fruits. Cooling spices are turmeric, coriander and saffron. Skincare products made with the fruit and seeds of the Neem tree are also useful.

Greasy, oily skin indicates a kapha imbalance. Increase your exercise and follow the kapha eating plan. Useful herbs include calamus, cinnamon, cloves, dry ginger, trikatu formula and turmeric.

TIPS FOR BEAUTIFUL SKIN
- Begin the day with a glass of hot water containing a squeeze of lemon.
- Take a daily capsule of turmeric.
- Enjoy regular massage.
- Use Neem or sandalwood soap for bathing.
- For some natural colour, drink fresh carrot juice and eat cooked beetroot (beet).

urinary infections

Cystitis is one of the most common infections of the urinary tract, particularly in women. It is generally a bacterial infection and should always be treated straight away because of the risk of it spreading to the kidneys.

Cystitis is mainly a pitta condition because it burns and is inflamed and hot. Avoid hot foods and spices and use plenty of coriander (cilantro). Other remedies include aloe vera juice (contra-indicated in

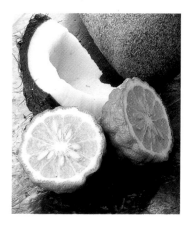

▲ Coconut and lime are recommended for pitta cystitis.

Tips for Treating Cystitis
• Avoid tea, coffee and alcoholic drinks.
• Personal hygiene is extremely important; always pull the toilet paper up and away from the body after defecation.
• Bathe with unperfumed oils and soaps until the infection has cleared.
• Coriander (cilantro), cumin and fennel tea is a good tonic. Use 1.5ml/¼ tsp of each herb per cup of boiling water.

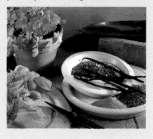

pregnancy), lime juice, coconut, pomegranate and sandalwood.

Kapha-type cystitis is accompanied by congestion and mucus in the urinary tract; the urine is often pale or clear. The treatments are cinnamon, trikatu combined with shilajit, gokshura and gokshuradi guggulu. Avoid salt, sugar and all dairy products.

In vata people, cystitis will tend to be less intense. Herbal remedies you can try include shilajit with bala, ashwagandha and shatavari.

index

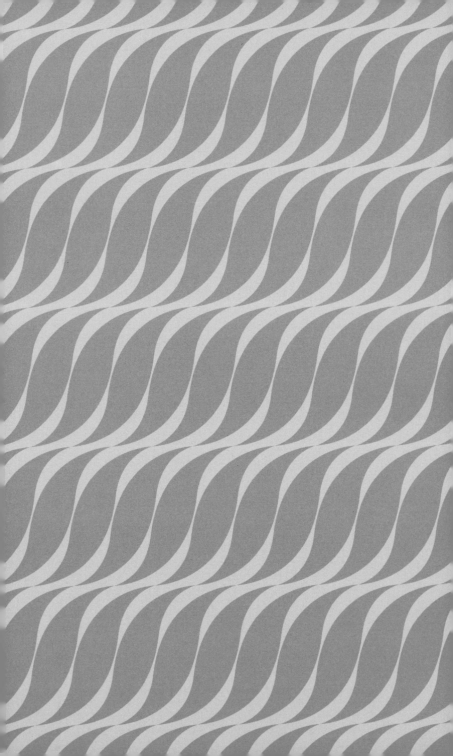